Fatma Chaker
Mohamed Derbel
Fatma Khanfir

Breastfeeding teaching kit

Fatma Chaker
Mohamed Derbel
Fatma Khanfir

Breastfeeding teaching kit

ScienciaScripts

Imprint
Any brand names and product names mentioned in this book are subject to trademark, brand or patent protection and are trademarks or registered trademarks of their respective holders. The use of brand names, product names, common names, trade names, product descriptions etc. even without a particular marking in this work is in no way to be construed to mean that such names may be regarded as unrestricted in respect of trademark and brand protection legislation and could thus be used by anyone.

Cover image: www.ingimage.com

This book is a translation from the original published under ISBN 978-620-6-71938-0.

Publisher:
Sciencia Scripts
is a trademark of
Dodo Books Indian Ocean Ltd. and OmniScriptum S.R.L publishing group

120 High Road, East Finchley, London, N2 9ED, United Kingdom
Str. Armeneasca 28/1, office 1, Chisinau MD-2012, Republic of Moldova, Europe
Managing Directors: Ieva Konstantinova, Victoria Ursu
info@omniscriptum.com

Printed at: see last page
ISBN: 978-620-8-60461-5

Contents

1 INTRODUCTION

Breastfeeding has benefits for babies, mothers and society. Early and exclusive breastfeeding is one of the crucial measures to ensure the survival of infants. According to the recommendations of the World Health Organisation (WHO) and the United Nations Children's Fund (UNICEF), it is recommended that children should start breastfeeding as soon as they are born and be exclusively breastfed for the first six months of life, and that AM should be extended up to the age of 2 by adding suitable complementary foods(1).

Globally, the prevalence of Exclusive Breastfeeding has risen from 40% in 2018 to 48% in August 2023, according to the WHO (2) . In 2012, the WHO set a global nutrition target to increase the rate exclusive breastfeeding at 6 months to at least 50% by 2025 and at least 70% by 2030 (1,3).

However, in Tunisia, this rate has not exceeded 13.5% from 2018 to November 2023 (4).

In response to this low prevalence, a number of factors need to be identified. Breastfeeding mothers face many complex challenges when breastfeeding. In addition, a lack of support from healthcare professionals is associated with the continuation of AM. Midwives are at the forefront of this issue. However, education about breastfeeding is often not taken into account in the training of healthcare professionals. Furthermore, in our practice, there is no normative approach to the management of post-partum AM (3).

What's more, according to the INPES (Institut National de Prévention et d'Education pour la Santé), the decline in breastfeeding is linked to a lack of knowledge, information, awareness and support for mothers, and a lack of self-confidence to breastfeed exclusively. In fact, women's confidence in breastfeeding plays a vital role in preventing early weaning. In other , any lack of self-confidence will lead to drop in breastfeeding rates(5,6).

For this reason, women should receive qualified breastfeeding support during pregnancy and post-partum from healthcare professionals(7). Done, it is necessary to improve their levels of knowledge and self-confidence in order to breastfeed successfully. These are factors that can be influenced by educational programmes (5).

This highlights the importance of improving management strategies focusing on information and education for breastfeeding women, particularly those most at risk from inadequate knowledge and low self-esteem, in order improve the knowledge base and AM rates to ensure the sustainability of this important practice.

Against this backdrop, we conducted a survey among a group of breastfeeding women with the following main objectives:

-Offer a specific breastfeeding teaching kit focusing on mothers' knowledge and sense of self-efficacy.

The secondary objectives were:

- To assess levels of breastfeeding knowledge and self-efficacy among early postpartum breastfeeding women.

-To explore the factors associated with breastfeeding knowledge and feelings of self-efficacy.

2 MATERIALS AND METHODS

1. *Methodology*

1) *Type of study*

The aim of this descriptive and analytical cross-sectional study was to assess breastfeeding women's knowledge and feelings of self-efficacy with regard to early postpartum breastfeeding, with a view to proposing a teaching kit.

2) Place and duration of study

The study took place in the early post-partum sector of the maternity ward of the Centre Hospitalier Universitaire (CHU) Hedi Chaker in Sfax.

Our study was carried out over a period of 1 month, from 20 January 2024 to 20 February 2024, to distribute and collect responses to the questionnaires.

3) Study population and sampling

-Target population: postpartum women who have given birth or are breastfeeding

- **Source population:** postpartum women in labour and breastfeeding women hospitalised in the maternity ward of CHU Hedi Chaker, Sfax.
- **Sample:** To carry out our study, we recruited 180 women from the post-partum departments of the CHU Hedi Chaker maternity hospital in Sfax.

To calculate the sample size, we used the following formula:

$$N=t^2 x\ p\ x\ (1-p)/m^2$$

- **t**: Confidence level (the typical value for the 95% confidence level will be 1.96)

- **p**: estimated proportion exclusive breastfeeding up to 6 months=13.5
- **m**: margin of error (generally set at 5%)

$$N=1.96^2 x\ 0.135\ x\ (1-0.135)/0.05=180$$

- **Sampling method:** non-probability convenience sampling

4) Inclusion criteria

Our study included: All breastfeeding mothers hospitalised in the early postpartum department of the CHU Hedi Chaker Sfax maternity hospital, regardless of delivery route, gestational age or parity, who were present at the time of the survey and who agreed to answer our questionnaire.

5) Non-inclusion criteria

We did not include :

- Women who refused to answer our questionnaire.

- The women were not admitted to the CHU Hedi Chaker Sfax post partum department.
- Women who have had a stillbirth, stillbirth or baby admitted to the neonatal unit.
- Women who have contraindications to breast-feeding as a form of medication.

6) Exclusion criteria

All incomplete responses were excluded from our study.

II. Evaluation method and data sources

1) *Measuring instruments and data collection*

To collect the data, we used an anonymous, self-administered, standardised questionnaire (Appendix A). It was chosen as the method of investigation to meet our objectives.

2) *Description of the questionnaire*

The questionnaire was administered in Arabic to make it easier to understand for some women with limited education. Illiterate participants were given a clear explanation using appropriate language and scales translated into Arabic and validated. The questionnaire was completed by the investigator herself (student midwife):

Our questionnaire is written in French and consists of 7 parts:

- **Socio-demographic data**

This section is designed to identify the woman giving birthage, origin, level of education, socio-economic level, occupation and habits harmful to health.

- **Obstetrical history and breastfeeding**

Gender, parity, previous breastfeeding, duration of previous breastfeeding, difficulties and level of satisfaction of women during previous breastfeeding experience.

- **Current pregnancy**

Antenatal monitoring, the person in charge of monitoring, mode and term delivery, number of children delivered and weight of the newborn.

- **Current breastfeeding experience**

Education and sources of information about breastfeeding, the intention to breastfeed, the expected duration and method of breastfeeding, initiation of breastfeeding, reasons for not breastfeeding, time of first latch, introduction of artificial milk and support at birth.

- **Assessment of breastfeeding knowledge among breastfeeding women**

Mothers' knowledge of was assessed using an Arabic version of the Breastfeeding Knowledge Questionnaire Short Form: BFQK-SF (BFKQ-FORM-A) (8).

The 16-item BFKQ-SF scale was translated and validated with Lebanese women in 2016 from the original 20-item English BFKQ.

The Arabic version has acceptable reliability, similar to the original instrument and covering various optimal breastfeeding practices with responses coded as 'true' or 'false'.

The BFKQ-Sf Arabic knowledge questionnaire on breastfeeding used several dimensions concerning information on the initiation of AM in the maternity hospital, factors that encourage the initiation of breastfeeding, signs of effective suckling, signs arousal of the newborn, as well as attitudes to adopt with regard to diet and rest. Other questions concerned the return home and the continuation of breastfeeding, as well as the benefits of breastfeeding.

True answers received one point each. Each participant was given a total of sixteen points to calculate a score. This score was used to classify the participants' level of knowledge into 4 groups(8) :

- Score <9: low.
- Score between 9 and 11: average.
- Score between 11 and 14: good.
- Score between 14 and 16: very good.

We also assessed women's knowledge of :

- Baby nutrition when a woman is at work or away from home
- Shelf life of breast milk at room temperature
- How to stop breastfeeding at the end of a feed
- Breastfeeding positions.

-Evaluation of women's self-efficacy with regard to breastfeeding

We used a short breastfeeding self-efficacy scale: BSES-SF (Breastfeeding Self-Efficacy-Scale-Short Form). This scale includes the mother's prescription on her ability to breastfeed. The scale was translated and validated in 2023 on a sample of mothers in the United Arab Emirates.

The BSES-SF is a unidimensional scale to be completed, with 14 items, organised into two domains, technical and intra-personal thoughts, presented in a positive manner and preceded by the phrase "I can always". It is scored on a Likert-type scale from 1 to 5, where 1 indicates 'strongly disagree' and 5 means 'strongly agree', with a minimum score of 14 and a maximum of 70 points. Higher scores indicate higher levels of breastfeeding self-efficacy. The total score was calculated by averaging the items answered, multiplying by 14 and rounding(6,9).

-Breastfeeding women's suggestions regarding the type and method of breastfeeding education

3) Data entry and analysis

The data were analysed using SPSS version 26 software (Statical Package for the Social Science) with a 95% confidence interval and significance index at p less than 0.05. The results were presented using Microsoft Office EXCEL version 2019:

-Descriptive statistics:For qualitative variables, we used frequencies and percentages. For quantitative variables, we used means and standard deviations.

-Analytical statistics : An analytical analysis using the ANOVA test was carried out with a significance level of 5% ($p < 0.05$). A 95% confidence interval is considered significant to study the relationships between the variables.

The results were presented in the form of graphs and tables.

III. ETHICAL CONSIDERATIONS Ethical considerations

Our study does not pose any ethical problems, as it does not affect either ethical principles or women's personal lives.

During our study, anonymity and confidentiality were respected.

We have obtained written authorisation from the head of the Maternity Department at the CHU Hedi Chaker Sfax.

While respecting the expectations and standards of the study, the results will only be used to answer our research question. (Appendix B)

3 RESULTS

I. <u>Presentation of the population</u>

The study population consisted of 180 women who met the inclusion criteria, had given birth at the CHU Hedi Chaker Sfax and recruited by convenience during the period from 20 January to 20 February 2024, through a questionnaire administered in the post-partum department.

II. RESULTS OF THE SURVEY <u>Results of the survey</u>

A. *Descriptive study*

1. Socio-demographic data

1.1. Age

The mean age was 31 years [18-44] and the standard deviation was 5.234. More than half of the women who gave birth (56.1%) were aged between 25 and 35 (Figure 1).

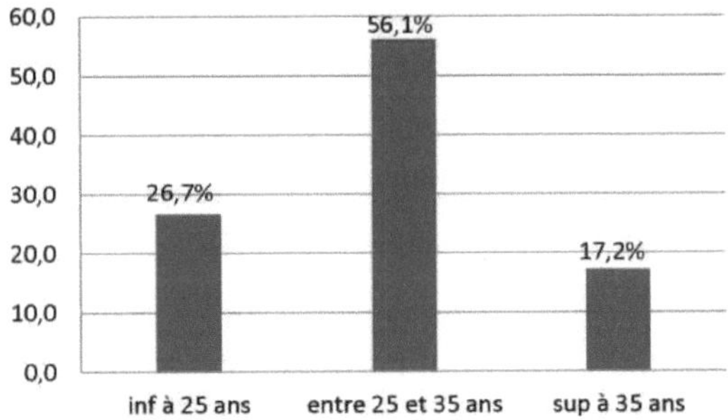

Figurei: Breakdown of women by age

1.2. Origin

In our population, 56% of the women were from rural areas and 44% were from urban areas (Figure 2).

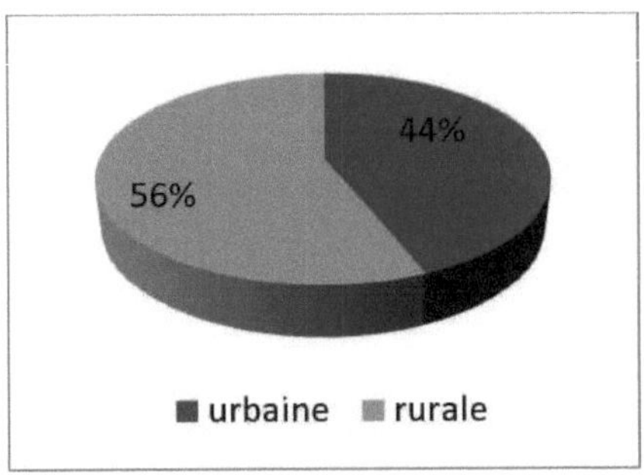

Figure 2: Breakdown of women by origin

1.3. Level of education

In our series, 53% of the women had continued their education up to secondary level (Figure 3).

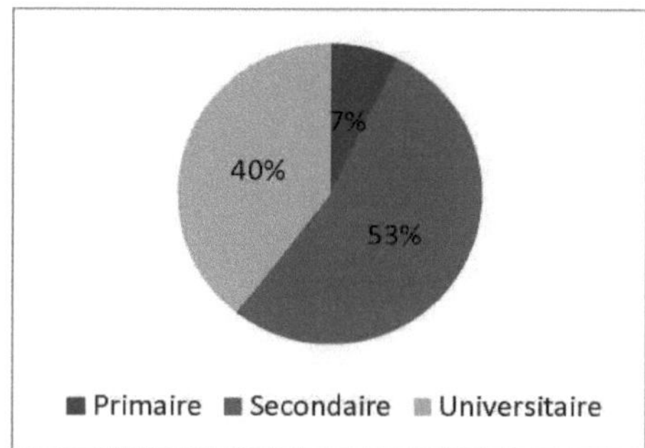

Figure 3: Breakdown of women by level of education

1.4. Socio-economic level

Of the women surveyed, 88% were from an average socio-economic background (fig. 4).

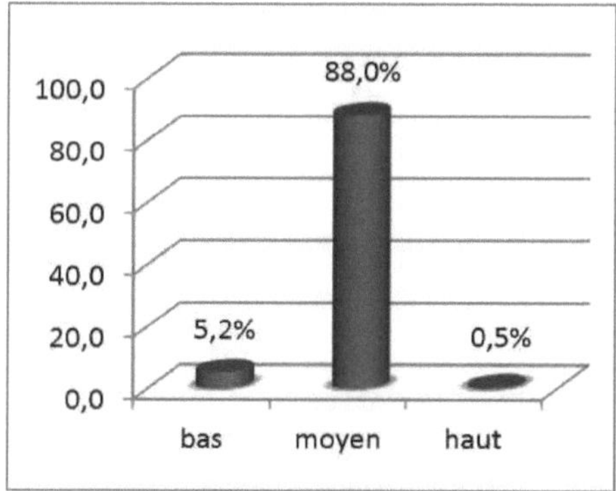

Figure 4: Breakdown of women by socio-economic level

1.5. Profession

Housewives accounted for 72% of the series, while 28% were employed (Figure 5).

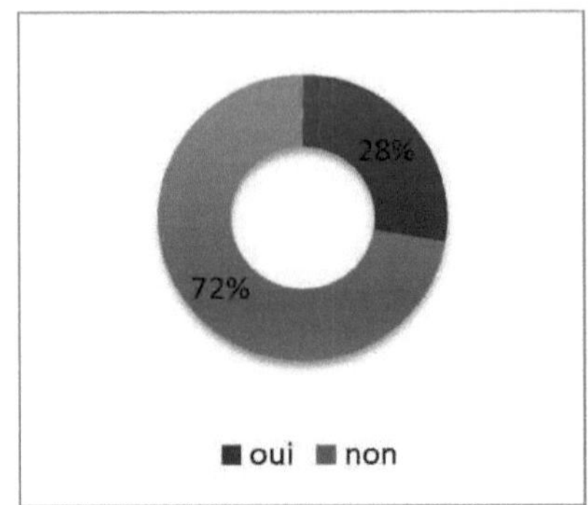

Figure 5: Breakdown of women by profession

1.6. Harmful habits

No harmful habits noted in 97% of the women, although 3% were smokers (Figure 6).

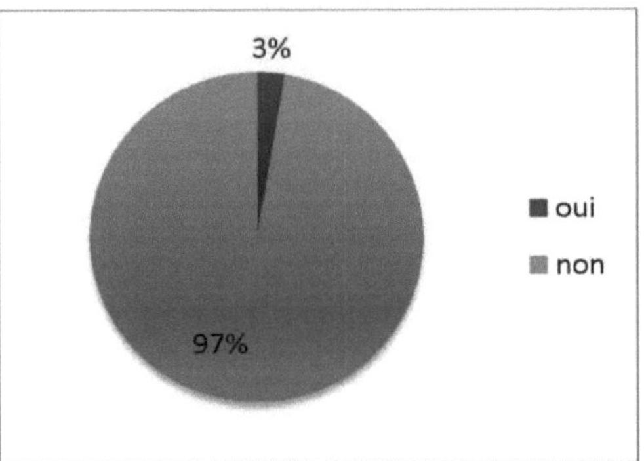

Figure 6: Breakdown of women by harmful habits

2. Obstetrical and breast-feeding history

2.1. Parity

The population was made up of 38.3% paucipares, 33.9% of primiparous and 27.8% multiparous (Figure 7).

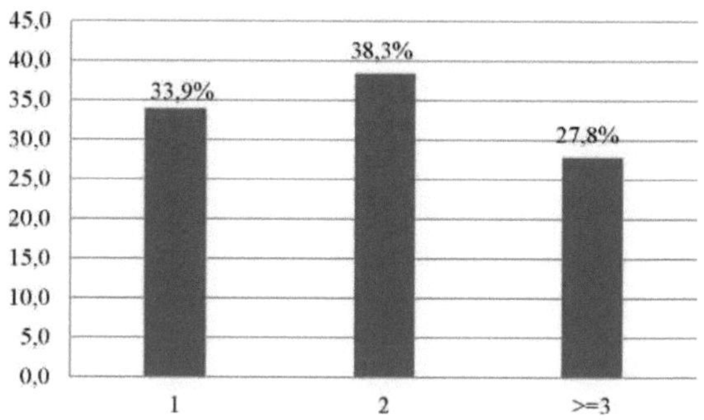

Figure 7: Breakdown of women by parity

2.2. History of breast-feeding

For patients who had already had live children, 96.6% of women breastfed, while 3.4% did not (Figure 8).

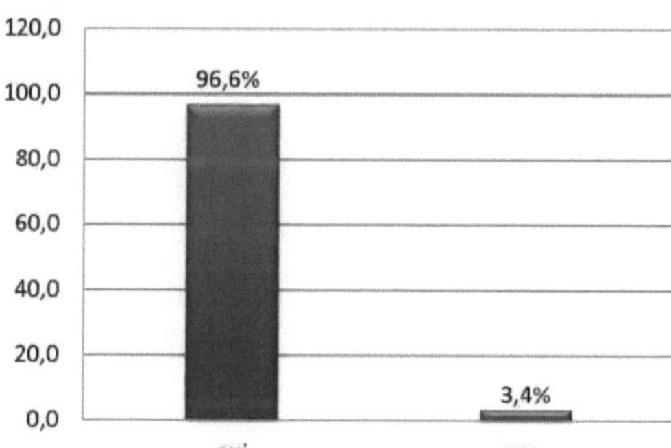

Figure 8: History of breast-feeding

2.3. Duration of previous breastfeeding

More than half of women breastfed their babies between 6 months and 1 year (53%) (Figure 9).

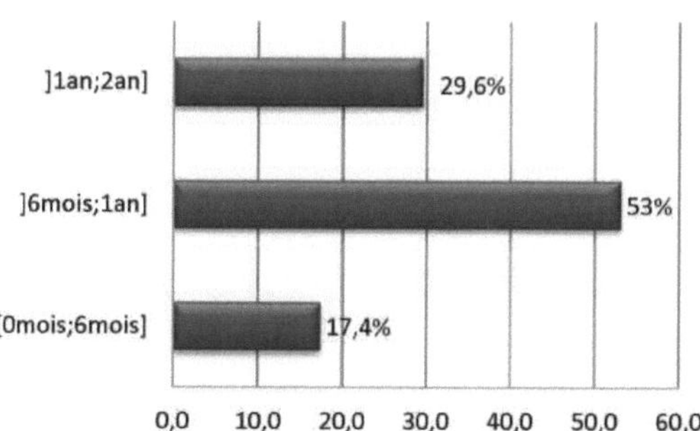

Figure 9: Duration of previous breastfeeding

2.4. Difficulties during previous breastfeeding experience

Previous difficulties were reported by 88 women (73.9% of women with breastfeeding experience). The most common difficulty was insufficient milk (22.7%) (Figure 10).

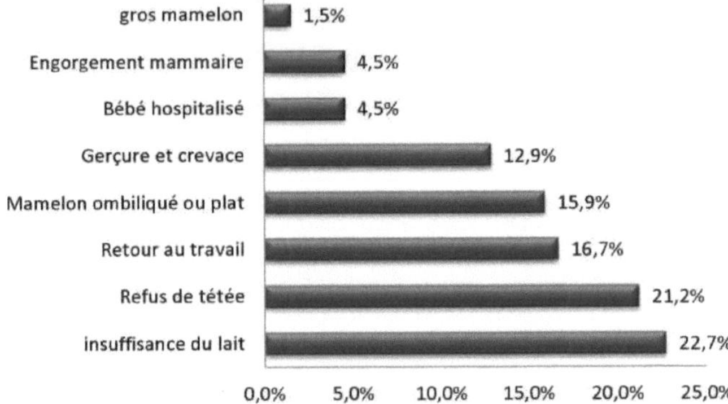

Figure 10: Obstacles to previous breastfeeding experience

2.5. Women's level of satisfaction with their breastfeeding experience previous

Women who were moderately satisfied with their breastfeeding experiences represented 68.7% of the population (Figure 11).

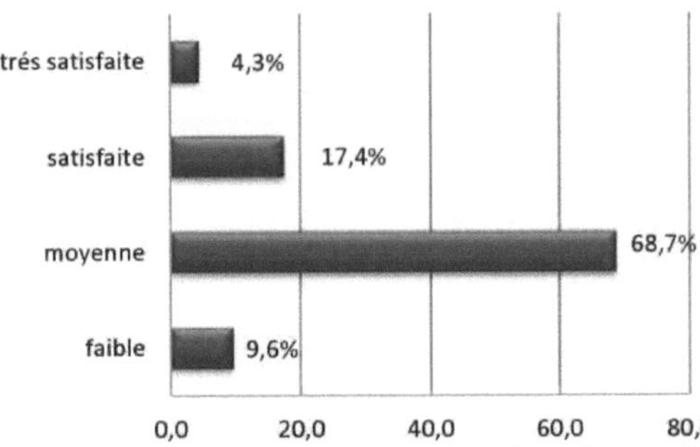

Figure 11: Women's level of satisfaction with previous breastfeeding experience

3. Current pregnancy

3.1. Antenatal care

In our study, 93% of women had monitored their pregnancies (Figure 12).

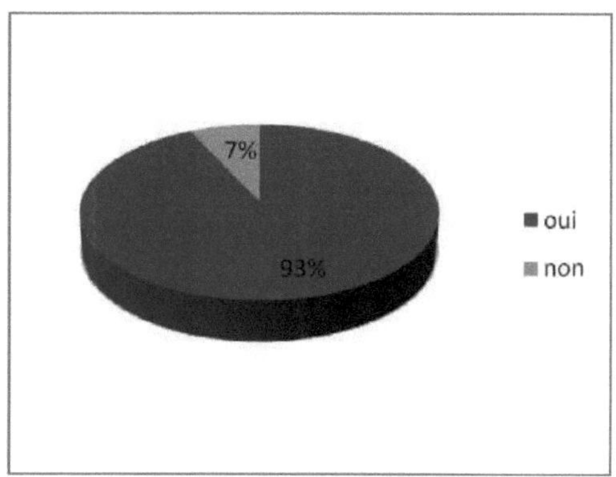

Figure 12: Antenatal care

3.2. Pregnancy coordinator :

More than half the women (60%) had followed their pregnancies with a gynaecologist (Figure 13).

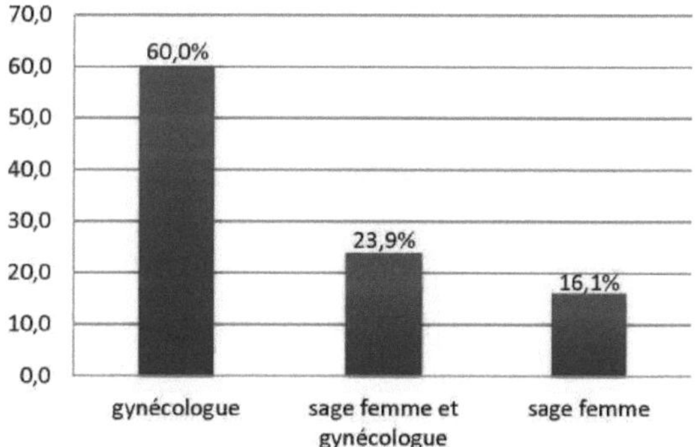

Figure 13: Monitoring manager

3.3. Delivery method

Women who had given birth vaginally represented 68% of the series (Figure 14).

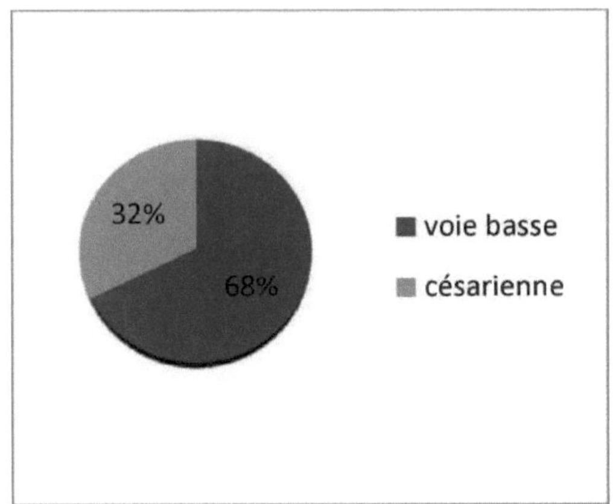

Figure 14: Delivery mode

3.4. Term of delivery

Premature delivery was noted in 8% of cases (Figure 15).

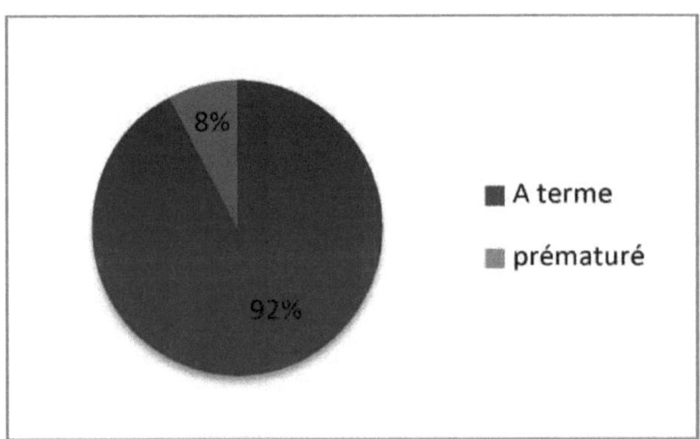

Figure 15: terme d'accouchement

3.5. Number of children delivered

Twin births accounted for 2.8% of cases (Figure 16).

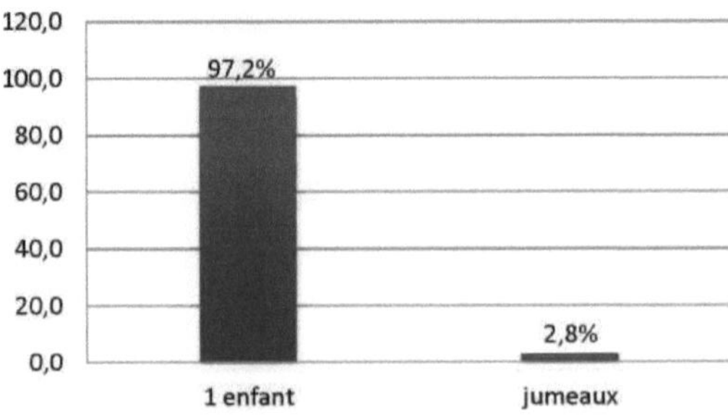

Figure 16: Number of babies delivered

3.6. Birth weight

Newborns with a birth weight of between 2,500g and 4,000g accounted for 85% of cases. (figure 17)

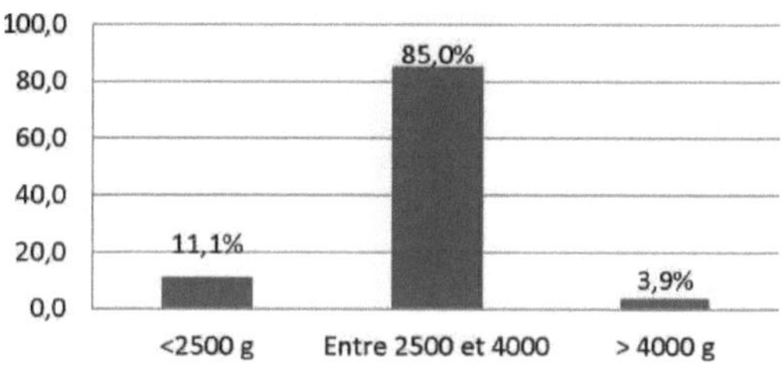

g

Figure 17: Birth weight

4. Current breastfeeding experience

4.1. Breastfeeding education

More than half the women (60%) had not received prenatal breastfeeding education (Figure 18).

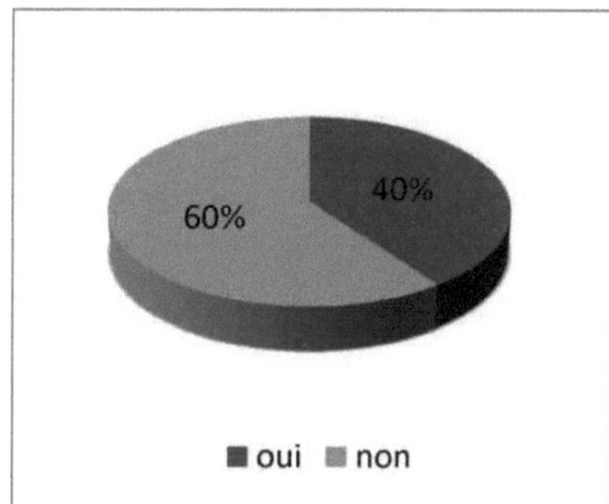

Figure 18: Breastfeeding education

4.2. Sources of information

In our population, the Internet was the main source of information about breastfeeding (34.2%). The midwife was the second source (28.4%). (Figure 19)

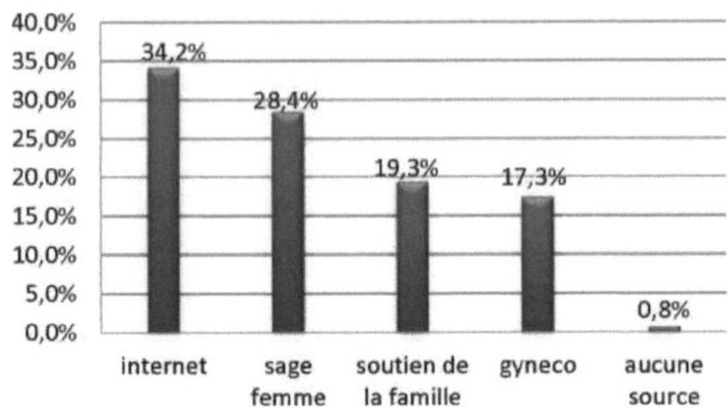

Figure 19: Sources of information on breastfeeding

4.3. Intention to breastfeed

In our study, no intention to breastfeed was observed in only 8% of cases. (figure 20)

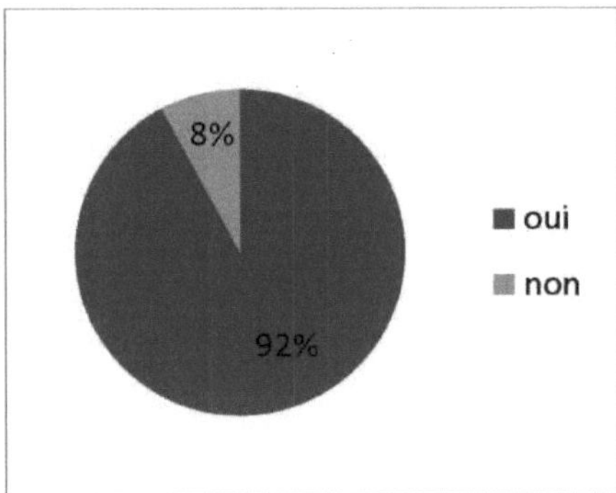

Figure 20: Intention to breastfeed

4.4. Planned breastfeeding method

Women who intended to breastfeed their babies exclusively accounted for 67% of cases. (figure 21)

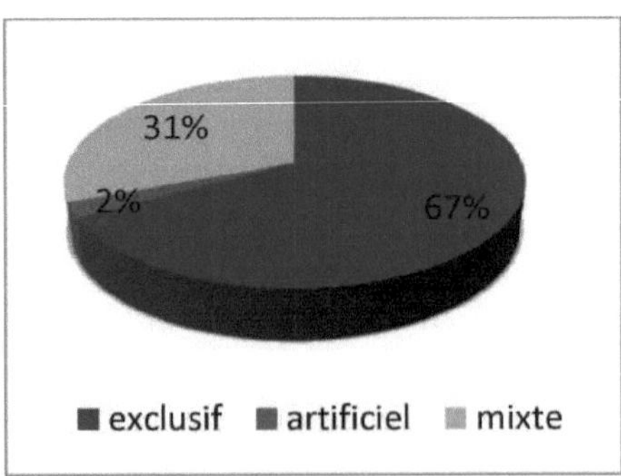

Figure 21: Planned breastfeeding method

4.5. Expected duration of breastfeeding

In our population, the expected duration of breastfeeding of more than 6 months was noted in 82.7% of cases. (figure 22)

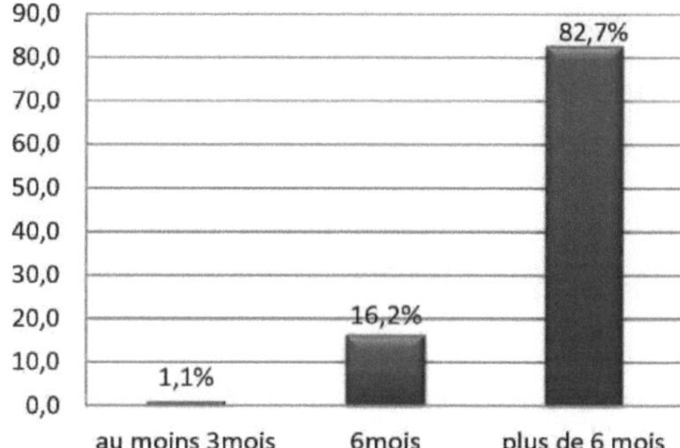

Figure 22: Expected duration of breastfeeding

4.6. Introduction to breastfeeding today

In our population, 87% of women had started breastfeeding their babies, while 13% had not (Figure 23).

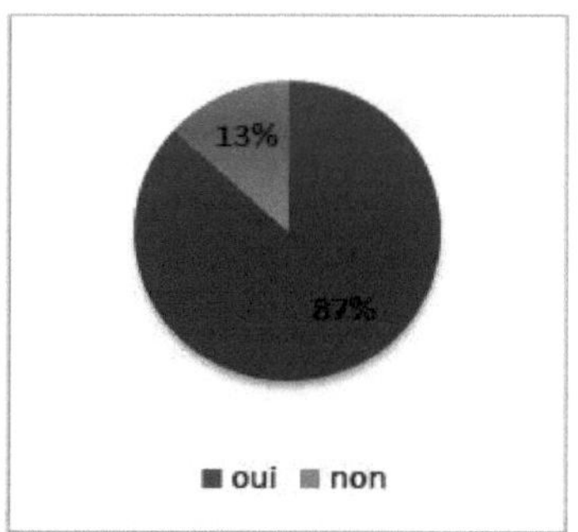

Figure 23: Introduction to breastfeeding today

4.7. Reason for not currently breastfeeding

Difficulties with current breastfeeding were encountered by 23 women (13%). The difficulties encountered are shown in Figure 24.

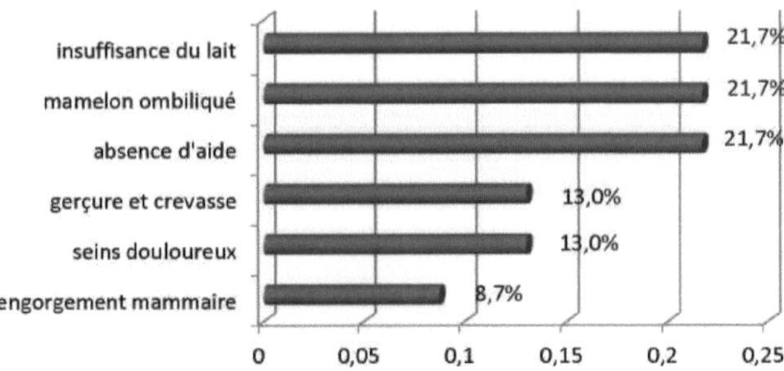

Figure 24: **Reasons for not currently breastfeeding**

4.8. Time for first breastfeeding

Almost half of the women had started breastfeeding 2 hours after giving birth (47.8%). The average time was 3.23 hours, with a standard deviation of 2.344 [4 - 16 hours]. (Figure 25)

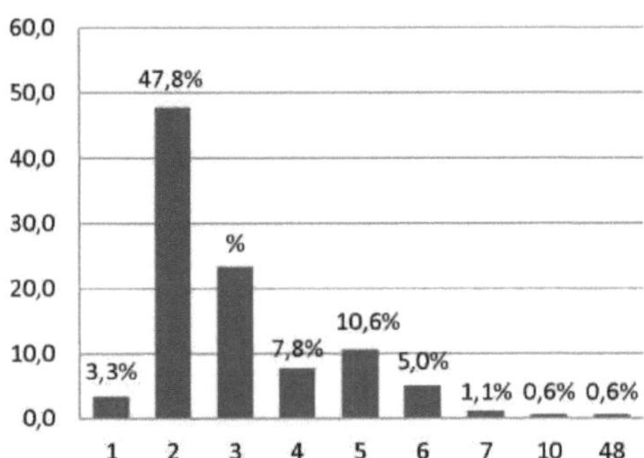

Figure 25: **Time of first breastfeeding**

4.9. Introduction of artificial milk

Artificial milk was introduced in 57% of cases (Figure 26).

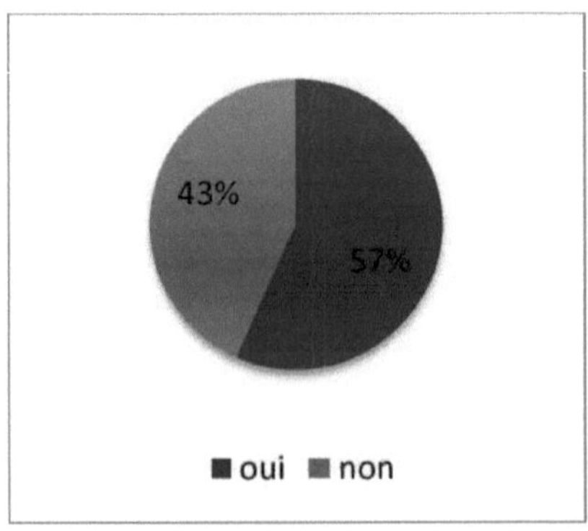

Figure 26: The introduction of artificial milki

4.10. Breastfeeding aid

Around 23% had received help at birth, while 71% had found no help at all. (Figure 27)

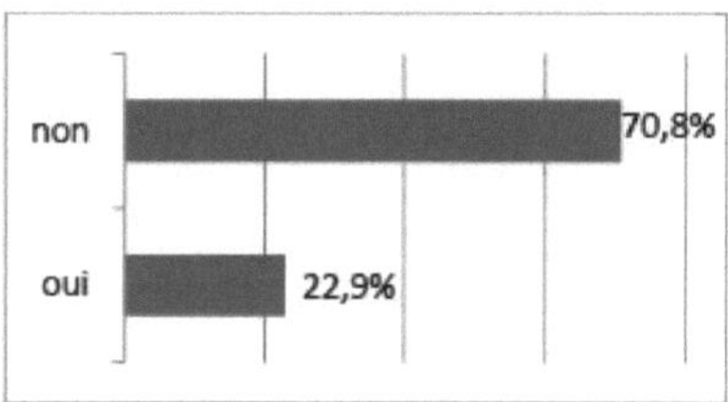

Figure 27: Breastfeeding aid

5. Women's knowledge of breastfeeding

5.1. Women's breastfeeding knowledge scores

In our population: (Figure 28)

J Half of the women had a good knowledge score (50%).

J 19% of women had an average knowledge score.

J 19% had a low knowledge score.

J 12% had a very good knowledge score.

J scores averaged 10.91 and the standard deviation was 2.344.

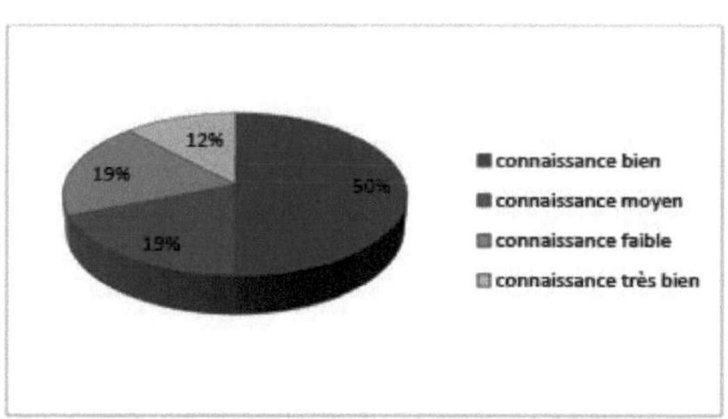

Figure 28: Class of knowledge scores

5.2. Feeding the baby if the woman is at work or away from home

Outside the home or at work, 56% of women said they would give their baby formula (Figure 29).

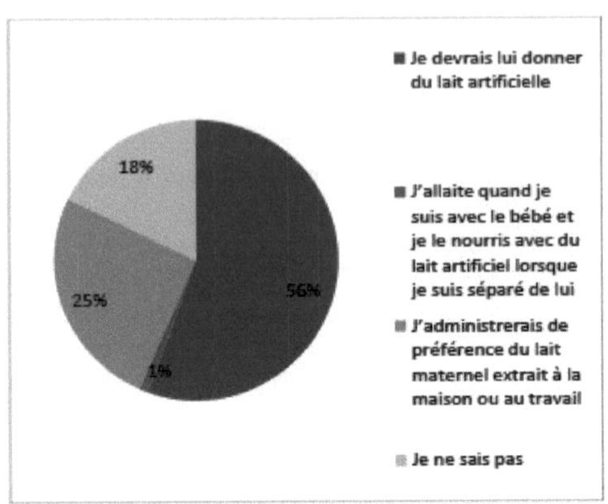

Figure 29: Baby nutrition when the woman is at work or away from home home

5.3. Shelf life of breast milk at room temperature

Only 13% of women knew that milk can be kept at room temperature for 4 hours. (figure 30)

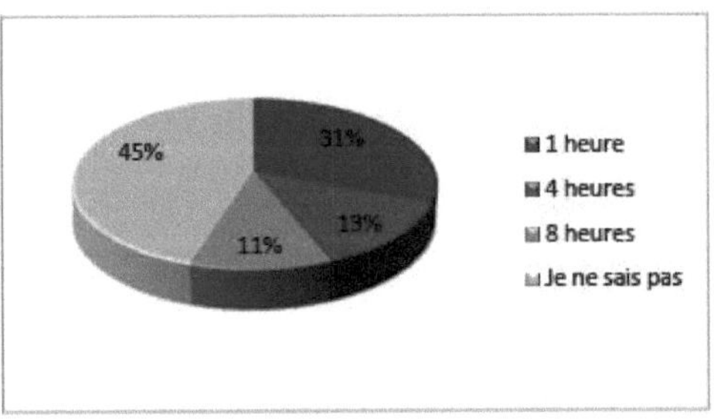

Figure 30: Shelf life of breast milk

5.4. How to stop breastfeeding at the end of a feed

In our population, only 37% of women were aware that breastfeeding had to be stopped by inserting a finger into the baby's mouth to release the nipple (Figure 31)

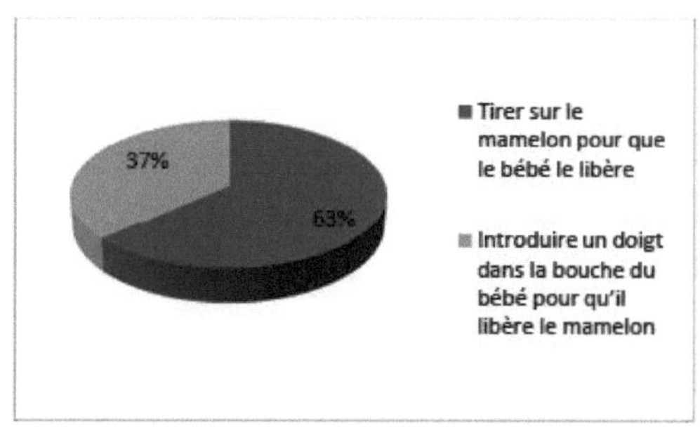

Figure 31: How to stop breastfeeding at the end of a feed

5.5 Breastfeeding positions

Patients were most familiar with the Madonna position (62.8%). (figure 32)

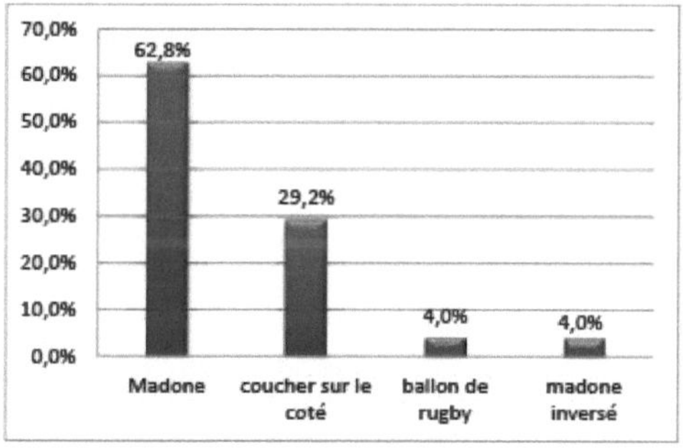

Figure 32: Breastfeeding positions

6. Women's self-efficacy score for breastfeeding

ȷ In our population, the mean score was 50.59, with a minimum score of 25 and a maximum of 68.

ȷ The standard deviation was 8.507.

7. Breastfeeding mothers' suggestions for breastfeeding education

7.1. The breastfeeding education method

Group education was proposed by 62.6% of women, while individual education was proposed by 37.4% of women (Figure 33).

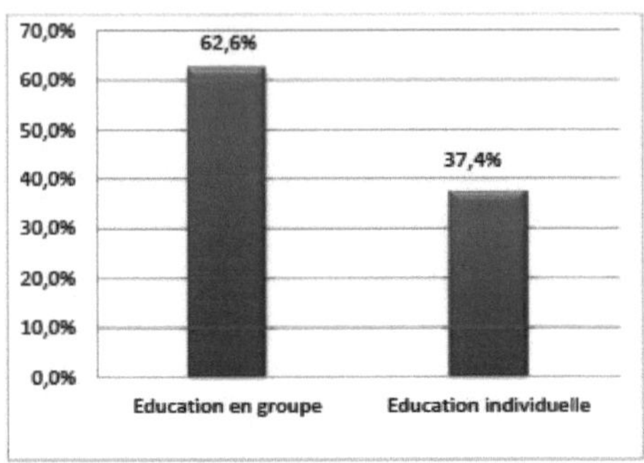

Figure 33: The breastfeeding education method

7.2. Type of breastfeeding education method

Assisted latching with postpartum assistance was the education method most suggested by women (23.2%). (figure34)

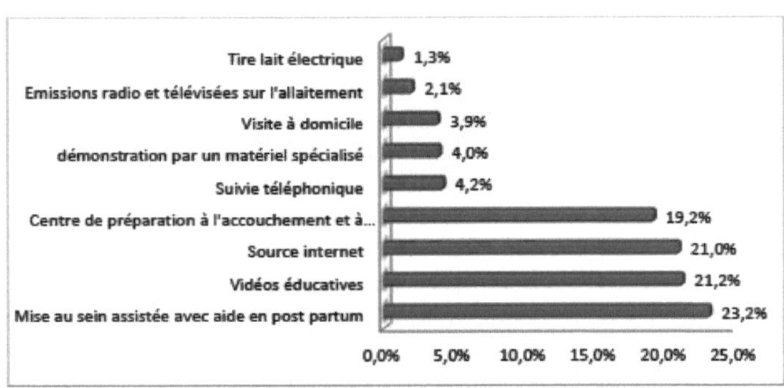

Figure 34: Type of education method

8. *Analytical study*

1. Factors associated with breastfeeding women's level of knowledge about breastfeeding

In the analytical study, the factors significantly associated with the knowledge score were age (**p=0.01**), level of education (**p=0.01**), sources of information (**p=0.03**) and the introduction of artificial milk (**p=0.03**).

Tableau I: Level knowledge of breastfeeding women according to socio-demographic data

Variables	Average knowledge	Standard	P (values)

			deviations	
Age	**Under 25**	10,63	2,385	
	Between 25 and 35 years old	11,32	2,135	**0,01**
	Over 35 years old	10	2,671	
Origin	**Urban**	11,15	2,214	
	Rural	10,71	2,434	0,2
Parity	**1**	11,30	2,201	
	2	10,62	2,408	0,2
	>=3	10,82	2,408	
Profession	**Yes**	10,52	2,393	
	No	11,05	2,317	0,1
Level of study	**Primary**	9,08	2,597	
	Secondary	10,94	2,379	**0,01**
	university	11,20	2,122	

Tableau II: **Knowledge levels of breastfeeding women according to current pregnancy data**

Variables		Average Knowledge	Standard deviations	P (values)
Antenatal care	**Yes**	10,87	2,350	
	No	11,31	2,323	0,5
Manager monitoring	**Gynaecologist**	10,91	2,417	
	Midwife	10,97	2,179	0,9
	Midwife and gynaecologist	10,86	2,315	

Tableau III: **Knowledge levels of breastfeeding women according to current breastfeeding data**

Variables		Average knowledge	Standard deviations	P (values)
Prenatal education	**Yes**	10,89	2,261	
	No	10,92	2,408	0,9
Sources of information	**Midwife**	11,05	2,341	
	gynaecologist	10,87	2,497	
	Internet	11,17	2,172	**0,03**
	family support	11,57	2,221	
	No source	8,00	1,000	

Method breastfeeding planned	Exclusive	11,02	2,344	
	Artificial	10,00	2,160	0,4
	Mixed	10,67	2,350	
Intention to breastfeed	Yes	10,98	2,340	0,2
	No	10,21	2,359	
Expected duration breastfeeding	Less than 6 months	8,00	1,932	
	6 months	10,69	2,163	0,1
	More than 6 months	10,97	2,654	
Breastfeeding previous	Yes	10,71	2,405	
	No	10,50	2,417	0,8
Introduction to breastfeeding	Yes	10,95	2,294	
	No	10,63	2,683	0,5
Introduction of artificial milk	Yes	10,49	2,367	**0,03**
	No	11,23	2,261	
Birth assistance and support	Yes	11,25	1,966	
	No	10,78	2,450	0,2

2. Factors associated with breastfeeding self-efficacy in breastfeeding women

In the analytical study, the factors significantly associated with the self-efficacy score were prenatal follow-up (**p=0.02**), breastfeeding experience (**p<0.001**), level of satisfaction with previous breastfeeding experience (**p<0.001**), assistance and support at birth (**p=0.04**) and planned breastfeeding method (**p=0.001**).

<u>Tableau IV:</u> Self-efficacy levels of breastfeeding women according to socio-demographic data

Variables		Average self-efficacy	Standard deviations	P (values)
Age	Under 25	51,54	9,107	
	Between 25 and 35 years old	50,51	8,510	0,5
	Over 35 years old	49,35	7,583	
	Urban	51,05	8,487	

Origin	Rural	50,23	8,549	0,5
Parity	1	51,05	9,989	
	2	50,65	8,062	0,7
	>=3	49,94	7,164	
Profession	Yes	50,36	7,845	
	No	50,68	8,776	0,8
Level of study	Primary	49,77	5,085	
	Secondary	49,79	7,731	0,2
	University	51,82	9,849	

Table V: Self-efficacy levels of breastfeeding women according to previous breastfeeding experience

Variables		Average self-efficacy	Standard deviations	P (values)
Breastfeeding experience	Good	54,78	5,493	
	average	50	6,743	**<0,001**
	low	43,67	11,113	
Level of satisfaction with the old experience	Low	42,62	10,206	
	Average	50,37	6,051	**<0,001**
	Satisfied	53,30	7,841	
	Very satisfied	50,48	5,727	

Table VI: Self-efficacy levels of breastfeeding women according to current pregnancy data

Variables		Average self-efficacy	Differences types	P (values)
Antenatal care	Yes	51,00	8,282	
	No	45,31	9,911	**0,02**
Person responsible for monitoring	Gynaecologist	50,70	8,358	
	Midwife	50,00	9,610	0,9
	Midwife and gynaecologist	50,70	8,285	
Number of children delivered	1	50,79	8,357	
	Twins	43,40	11,589	0,06
Birth weight	<2500g	50,25	8,372	
	Between 2500g and 4000g	50,84	8,429	0,3

	>4000g	46,00	10,520	

Table VII: Levels of self-efficacy in breastfeeding women according to current breastfeeding status

Variables		Average self-efficacy	Differences types	P (values)
Education in prenatal on breast-feeding maternal	**Yes**	51,06	7,312	0,5
	No	50,28	9,239	
Sources of information	**Midwife**	51,33	8,594	0,4
	gynaecologist	51,46	7,072	
	Internet	51,29	8,187	
	support from the family	51,77	8,827	
	No source	46,67	10,599	
Intention to breastfeeding	**Yes**	50,80	8,481	0,2
	No	48,07	8,731	
Birth assistance and support	**Yes**	51,29	8,922	**0,04**
	No	48,43	8,359	
Method planned breastfeeding	**Exclusive**	52,01	8,370	**0,001**
	Artificial	40,50	9,539	
	Mixed	50,55	7,816	

4 DISCUSSION

In this chapter, the results obtained are analysed on the basis of the scientific literature. It is important to remember that the main aim of the study was to exclusive breastfeeding, by proposing a teaching kit and specific educational programmes after identifying the key factors influencing breastfeeding mothers' knowledge and self-efficacy.

Recommendations and a conclusion are presented at the end of the study.

1. Characteristics of the population

The evaluation of knowledge and self-efficacy on AM was concerned, in our study, 180 breastfeeding women hospitalized in the early postpartum service at the CHU Hedi Chaker Sfax.

The average age of thc population was 31 and the standard deviation was 5.234. The largest proportion of the sample was made up of women aged between 25 and 35 (52.6%), 56% of whom were from rural areas. Of these participants, 88% had an average socio-economic level, 72% were housewives and more than half had a secondary education (53%). Of the 180 participants in the study, 38.3% were poor and 68% had given birth vaginally.

The internet was the most frequently used source of information (34.2%). Eighty per cent of women had started breastfeeding. Around 48% had started 2 hours after giving birth. The intention to breastfeed exclusively was noted in 67% of mothers. Despite this intention, 57% used artificial milk before leaving the maternity hospital, the main reason being insufficient breast milk (22.7%). Moreover, a study by Ayari et al. carried out in Tunis in 2022 also showed that 58.5% of women opted for co-education very early on and used artificial milk. The most frequently reported reason for this was the perception that there was not enough milk, which could be due a lack of information and therefore the risk of malnutrition for infants in the short or long term. It is for this reason that it would be imperative to provide breastfeeding women with even more support and to see a greater effort on the part of health professionals to help breastfeeding women, especially primiparous women, to overcome the difficulties encountered during breastfeeding(10).

2. Level of knowledge about breastfeeding

The results show that half of the respondents (50%) had a good knowledge score, 19%

had an average score, 19% had a low score and 12% had a very good score.

Several studies like ours have assessed breastfeeding women's knowledge levels using the BFKQ-SF. For example, in Spain in 2019, a study by Suárez-Cotelo et al. showed that more than half (55%) of women had a good level of knowledge, 25.5% had a neutral score and 19.5% had a low level (11). Moreover, according to Karimi et al, the knowledge scores of Iranian women were close to our study. Overall, 5%, 43.8%, 42.5% and 7.8% of mothers respectively had a low, average, good and very good level knowledge about breastfeeding(12).

Another study similar to ours in 2024 showed an average AOS knowledge score of 51% (13).

However, our results were inconsistent with those of a multicentre study carried out in 2017 among women hospitalised in 5 maternity and neonatology centres in Tunisia: Sfax, Sousse, Monastir and the Military Hospitals of Tunis and Mahdia. The majority of women (85.7%) had good knowledge of AOS(14). In this national survey, multiparous women had higher scores than primiparous women (p=0.018), whereas in the present study, the correlation was not significant with parity. This correlation could explain the average levels of knowledge in our study, since the percentage of multiparous women was only 27.8% of our sample.

On the other hand, a study carried out in Tunisia by Ayari et al. in 2022(4) showed that knowledge of breastfeeding was inadequate in 76.4% of cases. These inadequate levels of knowledge related in particular to the signs of effective suckling, the signs of arousal of the newborn, the rising of milk and the diet of the breastfeeding woman. This is explained by the mother's lack of professional activity.

3. Factors associated with breastfeeding women's level of knowledge about breastfeeding

factors that were significantly associated with the level of knowledge were: age **(p=0.01)**, level of education **(p=0.01)**, sources of information **(p=0.03)** and the introduction of artificial milk **(p=0.03).**

There was an association between the level of knowledge and the age of the participants **(p=0.01)**. Mothers aged between 25 and 35 had the highest average level of knowledge at 11.32, while those within the age range (under 25 and over 35) had the lowest average level of knowledge.

Similar results to our study, according to several authors, Al-Kordi et al, Al-Shehri et al and Al-Madani et al, in western Saudi Arabia (Saudi in 2014) found that mothers aged under 25 had less knowledge about breastfeeding and breastfed less than other women(15).

Similarly, another study conducted in Bamako, Mali in 2014 showed that there was a significant relationship between the level of knowledge of breastfeeding women and age, with a mean age 26.86± 6.44 **(p=0.01)** (16). However, other studies did not show a link between level of knowledge and age (p=0.09) (4).

These findings show that :

When mothers reach a certain age and become more mature, they become aware of the effects of AM for themselves and their children, especially if they have breastfed before.

The level of knowledge of breastfeeding mothers in our study was significantly associated with the level of education **(p=0.01).** Mothers with a university education had the highest average level of knowledge.

Our results were similar to those of a national survey conducted in 2022 at the maternity unit of the National Maternity and Neonatology Centre in Tunis. The latter showed that knowledge of the duration of exclusive breastfeeding was positively correlated with the mother's level of education; in fact, a high level of education is a factor regularly associated with a longer duration of AM(4). **These findings could be explained by the fact that 'emancipated', well-educated women seek to educate themselves in all matters relating to their health**.

However, in another study conducted in Tunisia, it appeared that mothers in developing countries breastfeed more and for longer the lower their level of education. Newborns of illiterate mothers were 1.9 times more likely to be breastfed than those whose mothers had seven years' education (4). The situation was different in industrialised countries. This phenomenon seems to correspond to the "popular model" described by sociologist Séverine Gojard in 2003 (17). This model was designed for women from working-class backgrounds with few qualifications. It was based on the predominance of the family as a source of information and advice. So breastfeeding in this model was represented as a natural act linked to the notion of pleasure for both mother and child.

Our results showed that breastfeeding mothers' levels of knowledge were significantly associated with sources of information **(p=0.04).** Breastfeeding mothers who had access mainly to their family circle first had an average knowledge of 11.57, and an average of 11.17 when they used the internet. An average of 11.05 was noted when the midwife was the source of information and 10.87 when the information was obtained from a gynaecologist.

All the studies on this subject gave a **very heterogeneous** picture of **the hierarchy of the different sources of information.** Some studies showed that the main source was family support, as was the case in Canada (33.9%), Brazil (59%) (14) and Tunisia in a survey conducted by Ayari et al. in 2022 at the Ariana Basic Healthcare Centre (4). Other studies showed that the main source was healthcare staff, as was the case in France (73.1%), Turkey (67.8%), Nigeria (88%) and Bamako (68.23%) (14).

In fact, the study by Blyth et al. in 2022 (4) showed a significant relationship between the information and degree of support received by healthcare professionals and the duration of breastfeeding. **This highlights the importance of fostering a positive sphere of influence around breastfeeding women because healthcare professionals have a poor role in informing women about AM. This leads us to question whether paramedical and medical staff are abandoning this role.**

This raises a number of questions: Is it the workload that forces them to shorten the consultation time for each pregnant woman? Or is the training of the staff themselves inadequate?

In addition, other results close to our study were reported by the African-American studies carried out by Duggan and Smith, in 2014 (18) at the University of California in San Francisco which showed that (90%) of women obtain medical and educational information breastfeeding and newborn feeding using social media and increased internet access to help overcome barriers and find social support.

In our study, there was a significant relationship between women's level of knowledge about breastfeeding and the introduction of artificial milk at birth **(p=0.03).** More than half the mothers introduced artificial milk (57%), and these had a low average level of knowledge (10.49). The reason most frequently given by mothers for substituting formula for breast milk insufficient milk, which was the most perceived obstacle in the post-partum period (21.7%). This remarkable result has been reported in several observations. Most often, this cause was associated with premature cessation of breastfeeding, between 2 and 6 weeks(19).

4. Breastfeeding women's sense of self-efficacy with regard to breastfeeding

The confidence of breastfeeding mothers is a key element of breastfeeding practices according to several studies carried out throughout the world. The mean BSES-SF score of our total population was 50.59, bearing in mind that the BSES-SF used in our study appears to be one of the most effective scales currently available for assessing mothers' confidence in breastfeeding and had a mean score of 14 to 70, with higher scores indicating higher levels of self-efficacy.

The results were deemed satisfactory in the present study, which may be due to the fact that these breastfeeding women had the desire to breastfeed. This desire is manifested by an energetic desire to breastfeed and by the mother's receptiveness to the pleasure of contact with her baby, or by the will to breastfeed, which is a faculty of the conscious mind for the decision to breastfeed and which is based on information such as self-knowledge and learning. These two psychological mechanisms, which are part of self-efficacy, are necessary for the breastfeeding project to succeed.

The scores in Tunisia in 2017, in a cohort study of breastfeeding women at the Farhat Hached University Hospital maternity hospital in the town of Sousse, were 44.88 ± 11.74 in mothers who were partially breastfeeding at 8 weeks postpartum, with a very low AME rate of 7.3%(19). The lack of confidence cited by mothers to justify supplementation or even replacement by formula milk was the impression that their milk was not sufficient to feed their baby. The same was true in Turkey in 2023. In fact, the mean score was very low on the first postpartum day (32.62 ± 8.82)(20).

However, the average self-efficacy score was higher in developed countries, particularly in 2022, in Brazil(21) when a biopsychosocial intervention strategy was used, which was the "kangaroo mother" method, or skin-to-skin contact between a premature or low-birth-weight baby and its mother or father from birth. The aim of this method was to encourage breastfeeding and to boost the mother's self-confidence in breastfeeding.

Also, in 2022 in Sweden (22), a study by Andreas et al. showed that breastfeeding mothers had good support for breastfeeding before leaving the maternity hospital, which resulted in high breastfeeding efficacy. Furthermore, self-efficacy improves the mother's adaptation to the infant, and this adaptation also reinforces the mother's self-efficacy with regard to breastfeeding.

5. Factors associated with breastfeeding self-efficacy in breastfeeding women

In the present study, a significant relationship was found between planned breastfeeding method and breastfeeding self-efficacy score **(p=0.001).** The mean breastfeeding self-efficacy score was significantly higher among mothers who breastfed exclusively, with 67% confident of continuing to breastfeed compared with 33% who were not confident of breastfeeding their babies without formula supplementation, given that the main cause was insufficient milk (21.7%), which also explains our exclusive breastfeeding result, with 92% intending breastfeed until 6 months of age.

Consistent with the vast literature, there was a statistically significant relationship between self-efficacy scores and continued breastfeeding. Thus, a low breastfeeding self-efficacy score correlated with bottle-feeding, a high breastfeeding self-efficacy score was linked to exclusive breastfeeding for a long period. In Tunisia, according to Sahli et al. in 2017 (19), the mean breastfeeding self-efficacy score was significantly higher in mothers who exclusively breastfed than in mothers who partially breastfed or interrupted breastfeeding **(p=0.001).**

Furthermore, in Brazil, according to Souza et al. in 2022 (21), there was a significant relationship between the breastfeeding self-efficacy score **(p = 0.025)** and the rate exclusive breastfeeding at hospital discharge.

In our study, there was also a significant relationship between the self-efficacy score and previous positive experience of breastfeeding **(p=0.001)** and the level of satisfaction during the previous breastfeeding experience **(p=0.001),** which can be explained by the fact that breastfeeding was part of the woman's history, updating her own experiences. In addition, these mothers were aware of the difficulties and were able to overcome them. As a result, they had greater confidence in themselves and in their ability to breastfeed.

These results were similar to Bandura's studies in 2017, which showed that previous breastfeeding experiences **(p=0.02)** and satisfaction levels **(p=0.001)** were significantly associated with an increase in self-efficacy (19). Moreover, according to Bandura's theory of breastfeeding self-efficacy, the active experience of mastery was one of the most influential sources of belief self-efficacy, because it was based on personal mastery of the tasks to be accomplished. The more successful an individual is at experimenting with a given behaviour, the more likely they are to believe in their personal ability to perform the required behaviour. Success, when it wasn't too easy, reinforces the belief personal effectiveness, whereas failure reduces this feeling.

This shows that :

A good previous breastfeeding experience with a higher level of satisfaction reinforces the feeling of self-efficacy, a bad breastfeeding experience with many difficulties in breastfeeding reduces this feeling and encourages early weaning.

The results of our study showed that a mother who received post-partum support (22.9%) had greater breastfeeding self-efficacy **(p=0.04),** i.e. good breastfeeding support gives the mother greater breastfeeding self-efficacy**. This indicates that health professionals, caregivers and the family should target breastfeeding mothers' self-efficacy in order to improve breastfeeding rates**.

Similar studies carried out by Andreas et al. in 2022 at the Swedish University Hospital showed that appropriate breastfeeding support had a positive impact on breastfeeding mothers' confidence in encouraging breastfeeding **(p=0.01)**. (22)

These findings show that :

To improve breastfeeding, support programmes need to be put in place for breastfeeding women. In addition, breastfeeding support should be part of routine medical check-ups.

In our study, mean breastfeeding self-efficacy score was significantly higher in women who monitored their pregnancies **(p=0.02)**. This was similar a study carried out in France in 2015 at the maternity unit of the Jeanne-de-Flandre Hospital at Lille University Hospital, which showed that the mean self-efficacy score was significantly higher, especially in the groups of first-time breastfeeding mothers who attended antenatal education sessions **(p=0.004)**(23)**.**

This shows that :

Antenatal care and breastfeeding education sessions for the couple increase maternal confidence and reduce the risk of early weaning.

In our study, there was no significant relationship between birth weight and breastfeeding self-efficacy score **(p>0.05)**. On the other hand, in Brazil, studies by

Souza et al. in 2022 (21) showed a significant relationship between the weight of the newborn and the self-efficacy of breastfeeding mothers **(p=0.04)** since the study was carried out in a vulnerable group consisting of newborns with a birth weight of 1800g or less. This was not the case in our population, which comprised 85% of newborns weighing between 2500g and 4000g.

With regard to level of education, a Tunisian study conducted at Sousse hospital showed that there was a significant relationship between mean breastfeeding self-efficacy score and the mother's level of education **(p=0.02)** (19). In our population, the higher the level of education, the higher the self-efficacy score, but the relationship was not statistically significant **(p=0.2).** Studies have shown that higher levels of maternal education have been systematically associated with longer breastfeeding duration in developed countries, whereas in developing countries a negative association has been demonstrated (24).

6. Breastfeeding education methods

Early and exclusive breastfeeding is an important strategy for improving the health of mothers and children. However, the targets a long way from the WHO and UNICEF recommendations universal or near-universal AME up to 6 months, and this can be explained by the lack **of knowledge, information about breastfeeding, confidence in the ability to breastfeed and support for breastfeeding.**

This requires breastfeeding promotion strategies based on information and education for breastfeeding women most at risk from low knowledge and low self-esteem, should be put in place improve knowledge levels and improve breastfeeding rates.

In Geneva, the WHO and UNICEF proposed a joint declaration on **Ten Conditions for Successful Breastfeeding**. It aims to protect, encourage and support breastfeeding. It forms the basis of the international Baby-Friendly Hospital Initiative, launched in 1992. Its role is offer recognition to hospitals whose maternity departments have implemented the ten recommended conditions.

Thus, condition number 3, among the 10 WHO conditions, focused on breastfeeding education, i.e. public health programmes aimed at health education and knowledge about breastfeeding were therefore essential. In addition, these educational programmes were inexpensive and had a strong impact on infant and maternal health, such as audiovisual media, which could potentially increase breastfeeding compliance in the Arab world. In fact, they have a positive impact on the knowledge, attitudes, self-confidence and practices of breastfeeding among mothers in Arab countries, and therefore on increasing the initiation and duration of breastfeeding(25).

Moreover, in our study and thanks to the question at the end of our questionnaire, the women were able to suggest the types and modes of breastfeeding education methods in order improve their levels of knowledge and self-efficacy for successful practice. The most popular method of education was group education at (64.6%), and the most popular types of education method were assisted latching with post-partum help (23.2%), educational video (21.2%), internet source (21%), birth and breastfeeding preparation centre (19.2%).

These methods have proved effective in the field of breastfeeding. Indeed, the results of a study by Elden et al in 2022 showed that digital technologies and social media have improved access to healthcare provision, in particular the promotion of breastfeeding(26).

In fact, according to Alnasser et al in 2018, global evidence showed that mHealth (mobile Health) interventions given the widespread use of mobile phones significantly improve exclusive breastfeeding. Similarly, according to Dinour, another study conducted in 2022 (20) highlighted the fact that 57% of mothers used a mobile app to their infant's feeding, and that mothers who used mobile apps had a higher rate of exclusive breastfeeding. In addition, he found that the majority of mothers used the app to monitor different aspects of infant nutrition, such as the start and end times of breastfeeding, the total duration of breastfeeding, and the number and quantity of regular breastfeeds(27).

Furthermore, according to Öksüz , in 2021 (20), he studied the impact of WhatsApp-assisted breastfeeding support on breastfeeding outcomes. He found that **the average** breastfeeding **self-efficacy score** was significantly **higher** in the experimental group than in the control group up to the second month. Also, according to Wu et al. in 2020 (20), a study evaluating the effectiveness of using "WeChat", one of the main social networking platforms in China, support breastfeeding, found that the breastfeeding rate was significantly higher in the experimental group (81.1%) than in the control group (63.3%) between 0 and 1 month after birth. Based on these results, it can be concluded that the breastfeeding training programme based on a mobile application enables mothers to prevent and resolve breastfeeding problems by obtaining the right information.

Furthermore, according to Wong and colleagues in 2021 (20), a meta-analysis found that theory-based, multi-component breastfeeding interventions of at least three sessions, through both face-to-face training and telephone follow-up during the antenatal and postnatal period, could be beneficial in improving breastfeeding.

7. Strengths and weaknesses

1. Highlights

In our study, the sample size was representative (180 breastfeeding women) which reflects the properties of our target population with a high degree of accuracy and therefore generalisation of the results is possible.

We also used scales that have been translated into Arabic and validated. These scales were a source of information and knowledge about the benefits of breastfeeding, and reinforced the feeling of self-efficacy in some breastfeeding women.

In addition, our study demonstrated the effectiveness of these two scales (BFQK-SF and BFSE-SF) in identifying mothers at risk stopping breastfeeding. Maternity care staff could use these two scales during the maternity stay assess levels of knowledge and self-efficacy with regard to breastfeeding before discharge.

In addition, with regard to the level of study, not only did we describe the population and identify the hypotheses, but we also studied the risk factors influencing levels of knowledge and feelings of self-efficacy, which enabled us to propose a teaching kit improve the rate exclusive breastfeeding up to 6 months, as recommended by the HAS and WHO.

This study also enabled us to find out the expectations and priority requests of patients hospitalised in the maternity department of CHU Hedi Chaker Sfax concerning breastfeeding.

2. Weak points

Our study has certain limitations, the main one being the way in which the participants were recruited; it was a non-random selection. In addition, the participants were selected from a single university hospital rather than several centres.

Also, the duration of the study was short at 1 month because of time constraints, which can make it difficult to gain an in-depth understanding of the factors associated with the level of knowledge and self-efficacy, which may bias the results.

8. Recommendations

The WHO and UNICEF have adopted a joint statement entitled "Ten conditions for successful breastfeeding"(28) (Appendix C). These are aimed at health services, whose role is decisive in encouraging breastfeeding, and indicate the best practices to be used.

All establishments providing maternity and newborn care should :

1- Adopt a written breastfeeding policy that is systematically communicated to all healthcare staff.

2- Give all healthcare staff the skills they need to implement this policy.

3- To inform all pregnant women about the benefits of breastfeeding and how to practise it.

4- Help mothers to start breastfeeding their children within half an hour of birth.

5- Show mothers how breastfeed and maintain lactation even if they are separated from their infants.

6- Do not give newborns any food or drink other than breast milk, unless medically indicated.

7 -. - Leave the child with its mother 24 hours a day.

8 -1- Encourage breastfeeding at the child's request.

9 - i- Do not give breast-fed children artificial teats or dummies.

10 -- Encourage the formation of breastfeeding support associations and refer mothers to them as soon as they leave hospital or clinic.

In addition, establishments should refuse to accept batches of breast-milk substitutes, feeding bottles or teats, either free of charge or at a reduced price.

Many countries are following these recommendations by developing strategies that combine :

- Training healthcare professionals support breastfeeding mothers
- Information campaigns
- The use of lactation consultants
- Support groups for breastfeeding mothers

The introduction of large-scale breastfeeding health education interventions not only influences the rate breastfeeding initiation, but also increases the duration of exclusive breastfeeding.

The introduction of large-scale breastfeeding health education interventions not only influences the rate breastfeeding initiation, but also increases the duration of exclusive breastfeeding.

So, in response to women's requests breastfeeding education, and since education through videos was in second place, we produced an educational video based on levels of knowledge measured by BFKQ and self-efficacy measured by BSES-SF, which represented an alternative for planning educational interventions since higher scores are linked to higher rates of AME. This video aimed answer women's questions and correct incorrect answers and false beliefs about breastfeeding, as well as to demonstrate the benefits of breast milk for mother and child in order improve the rate AME and its duration in Tunisia and come closer to the objectives and recommendations of the WHO and UNICEF.

But we hope to have good quality birth preparation and breastfeeding centres in our country, with home visits, telephone follow-ups and midwives specialising in post-partum support and assistance for women and their babies, as is the case in developed countries.

5 CONCLUSION

The main aim of this study was to produce a breastfeeding teaching kit. Its specific aim was to describe levels of knowledge and feelings of self-efficacy and to explore their associated factors.

The results of our study showed that breastfeeding women had very variable levels of knowledge and self-efficacy in relation to the various topics breastfeeding. Analytical analysis showed that there were certain factors associated with the level of knowledge and self-efficacy.

Prenatal follow-up, breastfeeding experience, level of satisfaction with previous breastfeeding experience, assistance and support at birth, and planned breastfeeding method are statistically associated with feelings of self-efficacy. The knowledge score is associated with level of education, age, sources of information and the introduction of artificial milk.

The participants in this study proposed an audio-visual support as a second breastfeeding teaching kit. Consequently, we developed an educational video as a proposal improve the level of knowledge and self-efficacy in breastfeeding, as well as the continuation of exclusive breastfeeding.

It would therefore be very interesting to improve and create new educational methods on the promotion of breastfeeding in order to ensure a better level of knowledge and a greater sense of self-efficacy, as well as to increase breastfeeding rate and achieve exclusive breastfeeding.

6 REFERENCES

1. World Health Organization [Internet]. 2018. breastfeeding.

2. Joint statement by the Executive Director of UNICEF and the Director-General of WHO on the occasion of World Breastfeeding Week [Internet]. 2023.

3. Dubik SD, Yirkyio E, Ebenezer KE. Breastfeeding in Primary Healthcare Setting: Evaluation of Nurses and Midwives Competencies, Training, Barriers and Satisfaction of Breastfeeding Educational Experiences in Northern Ghana. Clin Med Insights Pediatr. Jan 2021;15:117955652110107.

4. F. Ayari un,Y. Sdiri a,E. Cherifi a,S. Khemiri a,H. Chouroua _,M. Cheoura _,W. Belhajammar and,A. Karoui b.,MB Channoufi b.,S. Kacem a,R. Achour c. Niveau de connaissance des mères vis-à-vis de l'allaitement maternel à la sortie de la maternité souza. févr 2022;Tome 50(numéro 2):Pages 164-172.

5. Souza RCD, Wolkers PCB, Pereira LA, Romão RS, Medeiros ES, Ferreira DMDLM, et al. The possible mediating relationship promoted by the self-efficacy of breastfeeding associated with the Kangaroo Method on indicators of exclusive breastfeeding. J Pediatr (Rio J). Sept 2022;98(5):540-4.

6. Ahmed AH, Rojjanasrirat W. Breastfeeding Outcomes, Self-Efficacy, and Satisfaction Among Low-Income Women With Late-Preterm, Early-Term, and Full-Term Infants. J Obstet Gynecol Neonatal Nurs. Sept 2021;50(5):583-96.

7. Blixt I, Rosenblad AK, Axelsson O, Funkquist EL. Breastfeeding training improved healthcare professional's self-efficacy to provide evidence-based breastfeeding support: A pre-post intervention study. Midwifery. Oct 2023;125:103794.

8. Tamim H, Ghandour LA, Shamsedine L, Charafeddine L, Nasser F, Khalil Y, et al. Adaptation and Validation of the Arabic Version of the Infant Breastfeeding Knowledge Questionnaire among Lebanese Women. J Hum Lact. Nov 2016;32(4):682-8.

9. Radwan H, Fakhry R, Boateng GO, Metheny N, Bani Issa W, Faris ME, et al. Translation and Psychometric Evaluation of the Arabic Version of the Breastfeeding Self-Efficacy Scale-Short Form Among Women in the United Arab Emirates. J Hum Lact. Feb 2023;39(1):40-50.

10. F. Ben Slama,1 I. Ayari,2 F. Ouzini,3 O. Belhadj4 and N. Achour. World Health Organization. 2010. Exclusive breastfeeding and mixed breastfeeding: knowledge, attitudes and practices of first-time mothers.

11. Suárez-Cotelo MDC, Movilla-Fernández MJ, Pita-García P, Arias BF, Novío S. Breastfeeding knowledge and relation to prevalence. Rev Esc Enferm USP. 2019;53:e03433.

12. Karimi B, Zarei Sani M, Ghorbani R, Danai N. The Pregnant Mothers' Knowledge About Breastfeeding in Semnan, Iran. Middle East J Rehabil Health [Internet]. 17 June 2014 [cited 20 May 2024];1(1).

13. Korzeb B, Jabiry-Zieniewicz Z, Szpotanska-Sikorska M, Mazanowska N, Stelmach D, Knap-Wielgus W, et al. Level of Knowledge of Post-Transplant Women About Breastfeeding During Immunosuppression. Transplant Proc. May 2024;S0041134524001969.

14. Fatma GHARIANI ép. KHARRAT. CONNAISSANCES SUR L'ALLAITTERNEL, ETUDE MULTICENTRIQUE DEUX POPULATIONS : LES FEMMES HOSPITALISEES ET LE PERSONNEL PARAMEDICA [Internet]. [sfax]: Faculté de médecine de Sfax; 2017.

15. Shahbar A. Factors associated with breastfeeding in Western of Saudi Arabia. 2014;

16. Traoré M, Sangho H, Camara Diagne M, Faye A, Sidibé A, Koné K, et al. Factors associated with exclusive breastfeeding among mothers of 24-month-old children in Bamako: Santé Publique. 15 March 2014;Vol. 26(2):259-65.

17. Gojard S. L'allaitement, une norme sociale. Spirale. 2003;27(3):133-7.

18. Asiodu IV, Waters CM, Dailey DE, Lee KA, Lyndon A. Breastfeeding and Use of Social Media Among First-Time African American Mothers. J Obstet Gynecol Neonatal Nurs. March 2015;44(2):268-78.

19. Sahli J, Manel M, Dahmène K, Zedini C, Mtiraoui A, Ajmi T. Breastfeeding Selfefficacy and Breastfeeding Outcomes among Tunisian Mothers Delivering in a University Hospital in Sousse (Tunisia). Adv Res. 10 Jan 2017;12(1):1-11.

20. Acar Z, §ahin N. Development of a mobile application-based breastfeeding program and evaluation of its effectiveness. J Pediatr Nurs. Jan 2024;74:51-60.

21. Souza RCD, Wolkers PCB, Pereira LA, Romão RS, Medeiros ES, Ferreira DMDLM, et al. The possible mediating relationship promoted by the self-efficacy of breastfeeding associated with the Kangaroo Method on indicators of exclusive breastfeeding. J Pediatr (Rio J). Sept 2022;98(5):540-4.

22. Rosenblad AK, Funkquist EL. Self-efficacy in breastfeeding predicts how mothers perceive their preterm infant's state-regulation. Int Breastfeed J. Dec 2022;17(1):44.

23. Dégrange M, Delebarre M, Turck D, Mestdagh B, Storme L, Deruelle P, et al. Do confident mothers breastfeed their newborns longer? Arch Pédiatrie. July 2015;22(7):708-17.

24. Prandi Perrone RA. Self-efficacy in nursing mothers of premature infants. Rev INFAD Psicol Int J Dev Educ Psychol. August 3, 2021;1(1):363-72.

25. SINTE-PAGNOTTA, Lydie. Is pregnant women's level of knowledge about breastfeeding sufficient to meet the World Health Organisation's recommendations on infant feeding? At CHU UCL NAMUR sites Dinant and Namur, 2020.

26. Enein BHA, Dodge E, Benajiba N, Mabry RM. Interventions and programmes to promote breastfeeding in Arabic-speaking countries: a scoping study. 2023;13.

27. Enein BHA, Dodge E, Benajiba N, Mabry RM. Interventions and programmes to promote breastfeeding in Arabic-speaking countries: a scoping study. 2023;15.

28. Free [Internet]. 2023. 10 CONDITIONS for successful breastfeeding.

7 APPENDICES

Appendix A: Questionnaire

Socio-demographic data :

ý **Age :** [18 ;25ans [[25ans ; 35ans[[35ans ; 45ans[ý

Origin : Urban

Level of study Primary Secondary University ý

Socio-economic level: Low Medium High

profession: yes no **Gestité:.........**

Living child Yes No

Harmful habits Yes No

> Obstetrical and breast-feeding history :

- **Parity:**□ primipare □paucipare □multipare
- **Did you breastfeed your babies during your previous pregnancies?**

□ Yes : if yes, how many months do you breastfeed ;

□ [Months ;6months] □]6months ;1year] □]1year ;2years]

□ No

- What obstacles have you encountered in your previous breastfeeding ?

□ Cracks and fissures

□ Back to work

□ Insufficient milk

□ Refusal to feed

□ Umbilical or flat nipple

□ Other

- **Breastfeeding experience:** □ Good □ Fair □ Poor
- **Level of satisfaction with previous breastfeeding experience ;**

□ Dissatisfied □ Not very satisfied □ Satisfied □ Very satisfied

> Current pregnancy :

- **Pregnancy follow-up :**
- **Person responsible for follow-up :**
- **Mode of delivery:** Q vaginal delivery Q Caesarean section
- **Term of delivery**: □ full term□ □ premature
- **Number of children delivered**: Щ □ 2 □ plus
- **Birth weight**: □ <2500g □ Between 2500g and 4000 □ >4000g

> Data on current breastfeeding :

- **Did you receive any prenatal breastfeeding education**: □ yes □ no
- **What source of information is used for breastfeeding education?**

□ gynaecologist

□ Midwife

□ Source of weather □ Family support and husband □ No source

- Planned breastfeeding method Q Exclusive □ Artificiei□ Mixed

- Expected duration of breastfeeding: □ At least 3 months □ 6 months □ More than 6 months

- Have you started breastfeeding your baby : □ yes □ no

- **If not, why not?**

□ chapped and cracked □ insufficient breast milk □ breast engorgement |- umbilicated nipple sore breasts]-] lack of help

- **Time for first breastfeeding :**
- **Have you introduced artificial milk?**

□ Yes □ No

- Did you receive support at birth to help you breastfeed your baby?

□ Yes □ No

> Women's knowledge of breastfeeding :

- Test the information on child nutrition :

	Questions	**True**	**Fake**
1	Breastfeeding plays a part in preventing postpartum haemorrhage		
2	breast-fed babies are less likely to suffer allergies and illnesses than formula-fed babies		
3	many mothers do not have enough milk to breastfeed their children		
4	If your breasts are small, you may not have enough milk to breastfeed your baby.		
5	The more the baby sucks, the more the quantity of milk increases		
6	Babies fed on breast milk are less susceptible to infections than children fed on formula milk		
7	If a mother has a cold or flu, she can usually continue to breastfeed her baby.		
8	You should not try breastfeed your baby if you are planning to return to work or school, as you will not be able to be with your baby.		

- Tick the right answer :

9 - The best food for newborns is :

□ breast milk □ breast milk and water□ powdered preparation for infants

10- do not breastfeed if :

□ Birth of a twin by Caesarean section |-I If you drink a lot of alcohol

11- the nipple of a breastfeeding mother becomes sore when :

□ The breastfeeding position is incorrect

□ The mother's skin colour is light

□ It was the first baby she had breastfed

12-When you're breastfeeding your baby, the best way to find out if he's drinking enough milk is :

□ Baby doesn't cry

□ He doesn't suck his hand after finishing his feed

□ 6 or more wet layers for 24 hours

13-When you are breastfeeding your baby :

□ You can recover your health more easily

□ You almost always put on weight

□ You may feel weak when you feed your baby

14-If you are breastfeeding your baby:

□ No one else can help you with the baby because you have to breastfeed.

□ This will take longer than if you were to give your baby formula milk.

□ It will be very difficult to feed the baby in public places

□ None of the above choices is correct

15-breast-feeding can cause :

□ Sagging breasts

□ The size of your breasts increases after you stop breastfeeding

□ There is no difference in the size and shape of the breasts

16-Breast-fed babies need :

□ Exclusive breastfeeding for the first four to six months of life

□ One bottle of powdered infant formula per day

□ A daily dose of water

- If you work or are away from home, how do you feed your baby?

□ I should give him artificial milk

□ I breastfeed when I'm with the baby and I feed him artificial milk when I'm separated from him.

□ I would prefer to administer breast milk extracted at home or at work

□ I don't know

- Breast milk stored at room temperature can be kept :

☐ 1h □ 4h [Jh Q I don't know

- To stop breastfeeding at the end of the feed:

□ Pull on the nipple to release it

□ Inserting a finger into the baby's mouth to release the nipple

- What position do you adopt when breastfeeding?

□ Madonna □ Inverted Madonna □ Rugby ballEJ Lying on side

> Women's self-efficacy with regard to breastfeeding :

- How self-confident are you? Please tick the appropriate box:

	Not completelyconfident	Not very confident	Confident at times	Confident	Very confident
I can always be sure that my baby is happy when he's being breastfed					
I can still breastfeed my baby without using formula like supplement					
I can always make sure that the baby is properly					
attached to the nipple during feeding					
I can still leave even if my baby cries					
I can always be satisfied with my breastfeeding experience					
I can always finish breastfeeding my baby on the first breast before he switches to the other					

breast.					
I can still meet my baby's breastfeeding needs					
I can manage the time devoted to breastfeeding					
I can always tell when my baby has finished feeding					
I can still maintain the desire to breastfeed					
I can always make breastfeeding fun					
I can still breastfeed comfortably in the presence of family members					
I can still manage breastfeeding as successfully as other health-related tasks					
I can still breastfeed my baby at every feed					

Women's proposal on :

-The breastfeeding education method :

- □ Group education
- □ Individual education

- Type of breastfeeding education method :

- □ Breastfeeding assisted by a post-partum midwife
- □ Educational videos
- □ Application on the internet
- □ Free announcements in the hospital
- □ Telephone follow-up
- □ Home visit
- □ Other :

Thank you for your participation

Appendix B: Head of department authorisation

Annex C: Ten conditions for successful breastfeeding set out by the WHO and UNICEF

by WHO and UNICEF

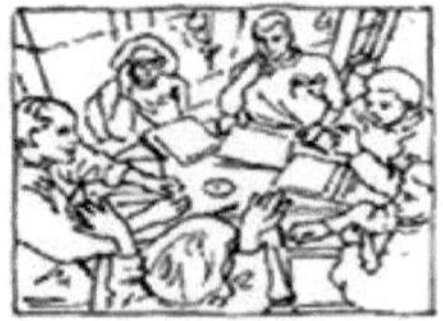

1. ***Adopt a written breastfeeding policy that is systematically communicated all healthcare staff.***

Assessment criteria

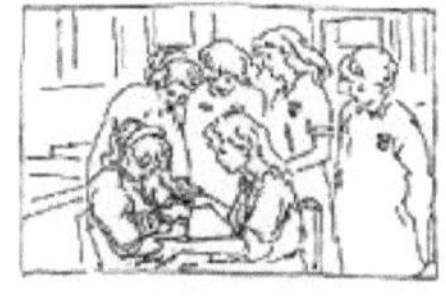

2. Give all healthcare staff the skills they need to implement this policy.

Assessment criteria

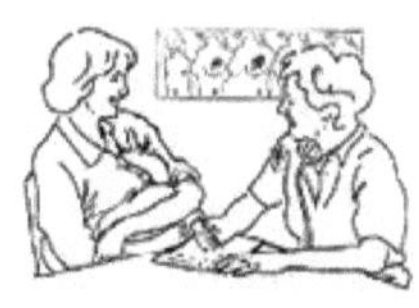

3. To inform all pregnant women about the benefits of breastfeeding and how to practise it.

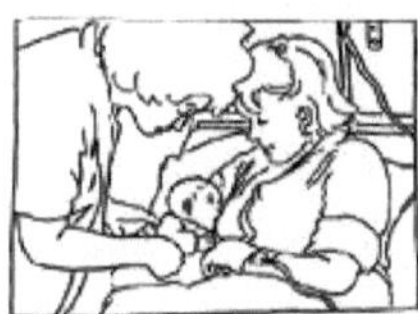

4. Help mothers to start breastfeeding their babies within an hour of birth.

Evaluation criteria

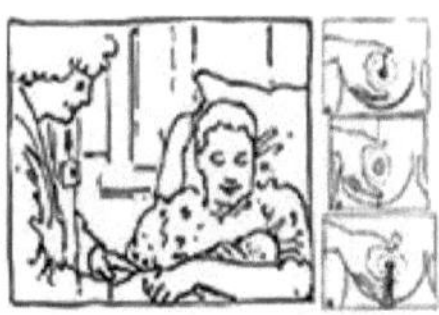

5. Show mothers how to breastfeed and how to maintain lactation, even if they are separated from their babies.

Evaluation criteria

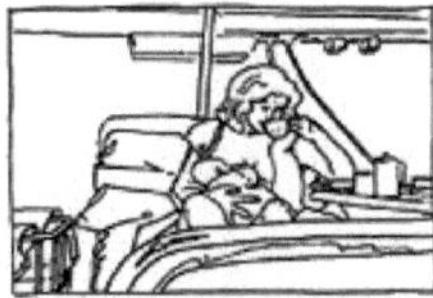

6. Do not give newborns any food or drink other than breast milk, unless medically indicated.

Evaluation criteria

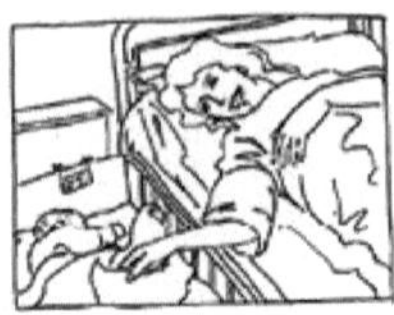

Practising mother-child cohabitation 24 hours a day.

Assessment

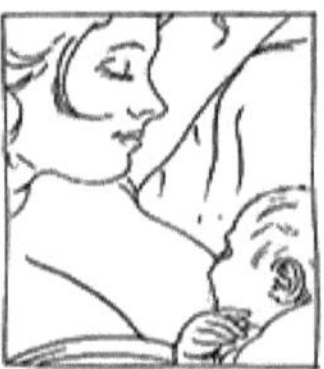

8. Encourage breastfeeding at the request of the child and the mother.

Evaluation criteria

C9. Do not give breast-fed children artificial teats or dummies.

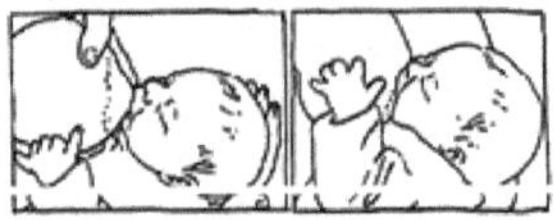

Evaluation criteria

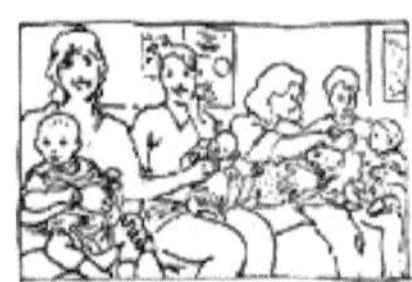

10. Encourage the formation of breastfeeding support associations and refer mothers to them as soon as they leave hospital or clinic.

Evaluation criteria

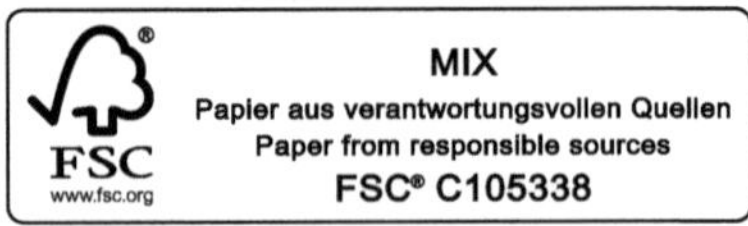

Printed by Books on Demand GmbH, Norderstedt / Germany